Trends in Oral Contraception

The Proceedings of a Special Symposium held at the XIth World
Congress on Fertility and Sterility, Dublin, June 1983

General Congress Editors:

R. F. Harrison,

W. Thompson and J. Bonnar

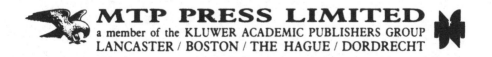

MTP PRESS LIMITED
a member of the KLUWER ACADEMIC PUBLISHERS GROUP
LANCASTER / BOSTON / THE HAGUE / DORDRECHT

Published in the UK and Europe by
MTP Press Limited
Falcon House
Lancaster, England

British Library Cataloguing in Publication Data

Trends in oral contraception.
1. Oral contraceptives—Congresses
I. Harrison, R. F. II. Bonnar, J.
III. Thompson, William, *1937-* . IV. World Congress on Fertility and Sterility (*11th: 1983: Dublin*)
613.9′432 RG137.5

ISBN 978-90-481-5802-7

Published in the USA by
MTP Press
A division of Kluwer Boston Inc
190 Old Derby Street
Hingham, MA 02043, USA

LCCN: 83-22257

Phototypesetting by Titus Wilson, Kendal
Printed in Great Britain by
Butler & Tanner Ltd, Frome and London

Contents

Manufacturer's Note:
The desogestrel/EE combination is marketed in different countries under the
following trade names: Marvelon, Microdiol, Marviol, Varnoline, Practil-21

List of Contributors

M. H. BRIGGS
Biological and Health Sciences
Deakin University
Victoria 3217
Australia

G. CULLBERG
KK. Ostra Sjukhuset
S-416 85 Goteborg
Sweden

F. R. HELLER
Laboratoire de Pharmacothérapie
Université Catholique de Louvain
53 Avenue E. Mourier
B-1200 Brussels
Belgium

E. KELLER
Universitäts-Frauenklinik
D-7400 Tübingen
Federal Republic of Germany

H. J. KLOOSTERBOER
Scientific Development Group
Organon International BV
PO Box 20
5340 BH Oss
The Netherlands

J. R. NEWTON
Department of Obstetrics and
  Gynaecology
Birmingham University Hospital
Edgbaston
Birmingham B15 2TG
UK

M. J. WEIJERS
Medical Research and
  Development Unit
Organon International BV
PO Box 20
5340 BH Oss
The Netherlands

General Congress Editors
J. BONNAR
Department of Obstetrics and
  Gynaecology
Trinity College
Dublin 2
Ireland

R. F. HARRISON
Department of Obstetrics and
  Gynaecology
Trinity College
Dublin 2
Ireland

W. THOMPSON
Department of Midwifery and
  Gynaecology
Queens University
Belfast
Belfast BT9 7AE
UK

The Special Symposium was Chaired by:
J. BONNAR, Department of Obstetrics and Gynaecology,
  Trinity College, Dublin 2, Ireland

A. KLOPPER, University Medical Buildings,
  Foresterhill, Aberdeen AB9 2ZD, UK

1
Serum glycosylated proteins as a measure of carbohydrate metabolism in users of oral contraceptives

H. J. KLOOSTERBOER, G. J. BRUINING, P. LIUKKO,
S. NUMMI and L. LUND

SUMMARY

Women using oral contraceptives may display minor alterations in carbohydrate metabolism. Using the oral glucose tolerance test (oGTT) it has been demonstrated that currently used low-dose combination pills induce an increase in the insulin response. In addition it has been suggested that during long-term use of low-dose combination pills glucose tolerances deteriorate. The oGTT is not performed under physiological conditions, and so it is questionable as to whether such a test truly reflects the glucose metabolic state. Moreover, the results are often influenced by factors such as stress and diet. The amount of glycosylated protein in serum is at present considered a good index of glucose homeostasis during the fourteen days preceding blood sampling.

A reliable method for the determination of serum glycosylated proteins, which allows assessment of carbohydrate metabolism under more physiological conditions than those found in the oGTT, has been developed in our laboratory.

This method was applied for the estimation of the effect of a new progestational compound, desogestrel, on carbohydrate metabolism. Glycosylated serum proteins, measured as the amount of hydroxymethylfurfural released per gram of protein, was estimated in (a) women receiving 0.125 mg desogestrel per day for 2 months and (b) women receiving the new oral contraceptive combination 0.150 mg desogestrel + 0.030 mg ethinyloestradiol (EE) for 3, 18 or 24 months.

It can be concluded from these studies that neither desogestrel alone nor the 150/30 combination of desogestrel and EE have any effect on carbohydrate metabolism.

INTRODUCTION

A decrease in the hormonal content of combined oral contraceptives (OCs) considerably reduces their effect on carbohydrate metabolism using the oral glucose tolerance test[1-3]. This test demonstrates a minor decrease in glucose tolerance and a small increase in insulin response in users of low-dose OCs. However, the results of an oral glucose tolerance test can be influenced by a number of factors such as stress and diet. This may partly explain the large variations found with a glucose loading test and makes it unsuitable for the detection of small alterations in carbohydrate metabolism as observed in OC users. Furthermore, the test is carried out with an amount of glucose that is normally not consumed in a single meal. It is therefore questionable whether the results of the glucose tolerance test truly reflect the actual glucose metabolic state.

Apart from the oral glucose tolerance test, the extent of glycosylation of haemoglobin (measured as per cent HbA_1) is used as an index of glucose control in diabetic patients[4]. The per cent HbA_1 may increase 2–3 fold in diabetic patients[4]. The value is already considerably increased in non-diabetic subjects with slightly impaired glucose tolerance[5]. Glycosylation of haemoglobin is a non-enzymatic process, which can occur with proteins in various tissues and with all blood proteins. In addition to HbA_1 the estimation of the level of glycosylated serum proteins is a good method for the assessment of glucose homeostasis[6]. The amount of glucose bound to serum proteins is determined by the time the proteins circulate in the blood and by the glucose concentration during that time. The value is 2–3 fold increased in diabetic patients.

In the present study, the glycosylation of serum proteins was measured in women receiving the new progestational compound desogestrel alone, and in women taking a new oral contraceptive combination containing 0.15 mg desogestrel and 0.03 mg ethinyloes-

0.15 mg levonorgestrel and 0.03 mg EE or from a control group without oral contraception.

MATERIALS AND METHODS

Young healthy women, aged 21–35 years, who had not taken hormonal medication for at least 2 months, participated in the studies. Blood samples were drawn after overnight fasting at the times indicated in the tables. Blood was allowed to clot for 45 min at room temperature and was subsequently centrifuged ($10^4\,N\,kg^{-1}$, 15 min) for preparation of serum. Serum was stored at $-20°C$ until use.

The following clinical studies were performed.

Desogestrel alone

A group of 10 women took one tablet containing 0.125 mg desogestrel per day for 2 months followed by 1 month without treatment.

Desogestrel + EE

Prospective comparative studies – Women received tablets containing either 0.15 mg desogestrel and 0.03 mg EE or 0.15 mg levonorgestrel and 0.03 mg EE. The treatment was started on the first day of the cycle. Each cycle consisted of 21 days of tablet taking followed by a 7-day tablet-free period. In one study the treatment period lasted 3 months and in the other 24 months. In both cases the treatment was followed by a control period of 2 months.

A retrospective study – The women came from an ordinary medical practice in the Netherlands. One group of women had taken the combination 0.15 mg desogestrel and 0.03 mg EE for 1.5 years and another comparable group of women had not used hormonal contraception.

Estimation of glycosylated proteins

The thiobarbituric assay was used for the estimation of the amount of glucose released as hydroxymethylfurfural (HMF) from the proteins

11

during hydrolysis at high temperatures. In comparison with other described methods[6,7] the procedure for hydrolysis of glucose from the proteins was modified with respect to three points. Firstly, hydrolysis was performed after removal of sialic acid; secondly, hydrolysis was carried out with acetic acid instead of oxalic acid; and thirdly, hydrolysis was done under anaerobic conditions. These alterations improved the sensitivity and reduced the variation of the method. The method will be described in detail elsewhere. The extent of glycosylation is expressed as μmol HMF released per gram of protein. For validation purposes, the method was also applied to haemolysates of diabetic patients on which an estimation of the % HbA_1 had been carried out by a standard chromatographic procedure. An excellent correlation was found between these methods.

RESULTS

The amount of HMF released per gram proteins in serum samples of 10 women receiving 0.125 mg desogestrel per day for 2 months was not influenced by treatment. The mean ($\pm$SD) pretreatment value was $0.79\pm0.11\,\mu$mol HMF $(g\ protein)^{-1}$; values after 1 and 2 months' treatment were 0.75 ± 0.13 and $0.75\pm0.17\,\mu$mol HMF $(g\ protein)^{-1}$, respectively. The post-treatment value was $0.7\pm0.15\,\mu$mol HMF $(g\ protein)^{-1}$.

Table 1 Mean ($\pm$SD) values of glycosylated serum proteins (in μmol HMF $(g\ protein)^{-1}$ in 10 women treated with 0.15 mg desogestrel + 0.03 mg EE or 0.15 mg levonorgestrel + EE for 3 months

Sample	Desogestrel + EE	Levonorgestrel + EE
Pretreatment	0.79±0.14	0.76±0.14
3 months' treatment	0.79±0.10	0.75±0.12
2 months' post treatment	0.78±0.14	0.70±0.14

Table 1 shows the results of a comparative study between two groups of women receiving 0.15 mg desogestrel and 0.03 mg EE or 0.15 mg levonorgestrel and 0.03 mg EE for 3 months. The amount of HMF per gram of protein was unchanged and no statistically significant difference was observed between the two groups. A similar result was found with both combinations after treatment for 2 years (Table 2).

Table 2 Mean (±SD) values of glycosylated serum proteins (in μmol HMF (g protein)$^{-1}$) in 10 women treated with 0.15 mg desogestrel + 0.03 mg EE or 0.15 mg levonorgestrel + 0.03 mg EE for 2 years

Sample	Desogestrel + EE	Levonorgestrel + EE
Pretreatment	1.05±0.14	0.97±0.10
3 months' treatment	1.14±0.16	1.03±0.09
6 months' treatment	1.07±0.12	1.01±0.10
12 months' treatment	1.05±0.10	0.96±0.12
18 months' treatment	0.97±0.13	0.86±0.12
24 months' treatment	0.99±0.16	0.85±0.10
2 months' post treatment	0.91±0.15	0.83±0.13

In the retrospective study it was found that treatment for 1.5 years with 0.15 mg desogestrel and 0.03 mg EE gave similar values for the extent of glycosylation of serum proteins to those observed in untreated controls: mean (±SD) values for glycosylated protein were $0.6\pm0.05\,\mu$mol HMF (g protein)$^{-1}$ in the treated group ($n = 27$) and $0.56\pm0.07\,\mu$mol HMF (g protein)$^{-1}$ in the controls ($n = 28$).

DISCUSSION

The estimation of glycosylated proteins as a measure for glucose homeostasis has a number of advantages over the generally used oral glucose tolerance test. The amount of glucose irreversibly bound to proteins is an indication of the status of carbohydrate metabolism over a longer period of time under physiological conditions.

The extent of glycosylation of serum proteins reflects carbohydrate metabolism in the one or two weeks before blood sampling since it is determined mainly by the half-life of albumin, which is 15 days.

13

In contrast, the oral glucose tolerance test is carried out with an unphysiological high glucose load and gives only an impression of glucose tolerance at any one moment. Glucose tolerance is influenced by several factors which may increase the variation of the test and makes it less reliable for detecting small alterations in carbohydrate metabolism. In our view the estimation of glycosylated proteins is a better alternative for assessing glucose homeostasis in pill users.

Small effects of low-dose combination pills on carbohydrate metabolism are observed using the oral glucose tolerance test. The test indicates a minor alteration in the glucose tolerance and a small increase in the insulin response[1-3,8]. The effects of progestogens alone at doses lower than those used in combined preparations on these variables are stronger than with low-dose OCs[9-11].

Desogestrel when tested for 2 months at a dose of 0.125 mg per day does not have an effect on the extent of glycosylation of serum proteins. The 150/30 combination of desogestrel + EE also does not influence the amount of glucose bound to serum proteins even after long-term use. Similar results were observed with the 150/30 levonorgestrel + EE combination. It can be concluded that glucose metabolism is not influenced by desogestrel alone or in combination with EE at the doses tested in the present study.

References

1. Wynn, V., Godsland, I., Nithyananthan, R., Adams, P. W., Melrose, J., Oakley, N. W. and Seed, M. (1979). Comparison of effects of different combined oral-contraceptive formulations on carbohydrate and lipid metabolism. *Lancet*, **1**, 1045
2. Briggs, M. H. (1979). Biochemical basis for the selection of oral contraceptives. *Int. J. Gynecol. Obstet.*, **16**, 509
3. Spellacy, W. N. (1982). Carbohydrate metabolism during treatment with estrogen, progestogen, and low-dose oral contraceptives. *Am. J. Obstet. Gynecol.*, **142**, 732
4. Abraham, E. C., Huff, T. A., Cope, N. D., Wilson, J. B. Jr., Bransome, E. D. and Huisman, T. H. J. (1978). Determination of the glycosylated hemoglobins (HbA₁) with a new microcolumn procedure. *Diabetes*, **27**, 931
5. Verrillo, A., de Teresa, A., Golia, R. and Nunziata, V. (1983). The relationship between glycosylated haemoglobin levels and various degrees of glucose intolerance. *Diabetologia*, **24**, 391
6. McFarland, K. F., Catalano, E. W., Day, J. F., Thorpe, S. R. and Baynes, J. W. (1979). Non-enzymatic glucosylation of serum proteins in diabetes mellitus. *Diabetes*, **28**, 1011
7. Yue, D. K., Morris, K., McLennan, S. and Turtle, J. R. (1980). Glycosylation of plasma protein and its relation to glycosylated hemoglobin in diabetes. *Diabetes*, **29**, 296

8. Vermeulen, A. and Thiery, M. (1982). Metabolic effects of the triphasic oral contraceptive Trigynon. *Contraception*, **26**, 505

9. Spellacy, W. N., Buhi, W. C. and Birk, S. A. (1981). Prospective studies of carbohydrate metabolism in 'normal' women using norgestrel for eighteen months. *Fertil. Steril.*, **35**, 167

10. Spellacy, W. N., Buhi, W. C. and Birk, S. A. (1976). Carbohydrate and lipid metabolic studies before and after one year of treatment with ethynodiol diacetate in 'normal' women. *Fertil. Steril.*, **27**, 900

11. Spellacy, W. N., Buhi, W. C. and Birk, S. A. (1975). Effects of norethindrone on carbohydrate and lipid metabolism. *Obstet. Gynecol.*, **46**, 560

2
Androgenic, oestrogenic and antioestrogenic effects of desogestrel and lynestrenol alone: effects on serum proteins, sex hormones and vaginal cytology

G. CULLBERG and L.-Å. MATTSSON

SUMMARY

Desogestrel (Dgl)/ ethinyloestradiol (Marvelon, Organon) has a pronounced increasing effect on sex hormone binding globulin (SHBG). This can be due to an oestrogenic effect of Dgl or lack of androgenicity. These possibilities were evaluated using the effects on serum proteins and vaginal cytology. 0.125, 0.250 and 0.500 mg Dgl daily was given orally in a randomized order to eight healthy fertile women and also, in comparison 5 mg lynestrenol (Lyn). Each treatment lasted 6 weeks. The methods used were electroimmunoassay for SHBG, ceruloplasmin, cortisol binding globulin (CBG), thyroxin binding globulin (TBG) and prealbumin, radioimmunoassay for 17β-oestradiol (E_2), testosterone and vaginal cytology as maturation value (MV). Results found indicated a dose-dependent depression of E_2, SHBG and MV. The correlation was however much stronger for Dgl dose versus SHBG decrease ($r=0.97$) than for E_2 decrease versus SHBG ($r=0.54$) indicating an *hepatocyte blocking effect* by Dgl rather than a lowered E_2-stimulation of SHBG production. No *androgenic effects* such as increases in prealbumin or depression of TBG were seen after Dgl but a small significant increase in prealbumin was found for Lyn. No *oestrogenic effects* such as increases in CBG, ceruloplasmin or MV were seen for Dgl or Lyn but an antioestrogenic effect on NV was seen.

INTRODUCTION

During the past 5 years it has been shown that some of the most widely used gestogens behave in many ways metabolically as androgens[1]. Epidemiological studies suggest that lipid patterns, for example low HDL cholesterol values are correlated with increased risk for coronary heart disease[2]. The androgenic side-effects of oral contraceptives such as weight gain, hirsutism and acne, are common causes of withdrawal.

It is thus important to find gestogens with less androgenicity. Starting from lynestrenol, the desogestrel was synthesized (Figure

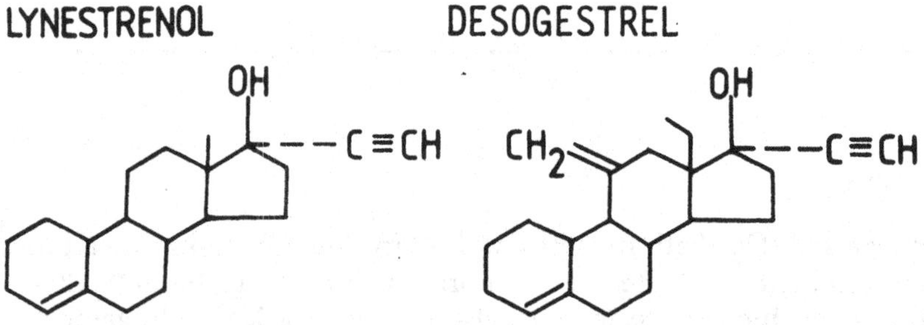

LYNESTRENOL   DESOGESTREL

Figure 1 Structural formulae of lynestrenol and desogestrel

1). When combined with ethinyloestradiol it appeared to be devoid of androgenicity in spite of being a 19-nor-testosterone derivate[3]. It allows increases in sex hormone binding globulin (SHBG) and HDL-cholesterol values in contrast to the other gonane, levonorgestrel. But interesting questions arise; does it have any oestrogenic, antioestrogenic or androgenic properties when given alone in comparison with, for example, lynestrenol?

To find out, we performed a study evaluating vaginal cytology and serum proteins from eight regularly menstruating women who were healthy apart from endometriosis. They had not taken any hormones during the last 3 months. A blood sample was taken before treatment.

18

The women were then given 0.125, 0.25 or 0.5 mg desogestrel and 5 mg lynestrenol in daily doses (Table 1). The treatments were given in a randomized order, i.e. one women starting with lynestrenol

Table 1 Examples of experimental protocol. The other four women had similar cycles of drug intake. Each treatment was taken for 6 weeks and samples taken at 0, 6, 12, 18 and 24 weeks

	Treatment*			
Patient	1	2	3	4
1	L	0.125 D	0.25 D	0.5 D
2	0.125 D	L	0.5 D	0.25 D
3	0.125 D	0.5 D	0.25 D	L
8	0.5 D	0.25 D	L	0.125 D

*Figures are mg taken daily.
D = Desogestrel; L = 5 mg lynestrenol.

and then going on with the desogestrel and another starting with desogestrel, etc. Each dose was given for 6 weeks without any treatment-free intervals.

Serum was analysed for SHBG, cortisol binding globulin (CBG), ceruloplasmin, thyroxin binding globulin (TBG) and prealbumin using electroimmunoassay according to Laurell[4]. Vaginal cytology was judged as maturation values, giving the percentage of superficial cells the multiplication factor 1.0 and adding an intermediate-cell percentage multiplied by 0.5. Serum oestradiol and testosterone were analysed with radioimmunoassay.

RESULTS AND DISCUSSION

When a synthetic oestrogen is given, the levels of SHBG, TBG, CBG and ceruloplasmin rise and the maturation value is increased while ovarian hormone production is sometimes stimulated and sometimes depressed, depending on the dosage and type of hormone. Androgens have the opposite effect on SHBG and TBG but have very little influence on CBG and ceruloplasmin. The prealbumin level is not influenced by oestrogens but is increased when an androgenic substance is given[3-5].

In the present study serum levels of oestradiol were significantly lowered in relation to the desogestrel dose except in two women during the 0.125 mg treatment (Figure 2). Testosterone levels were also lower during treatment with desogestrel but not with lynestrenol.

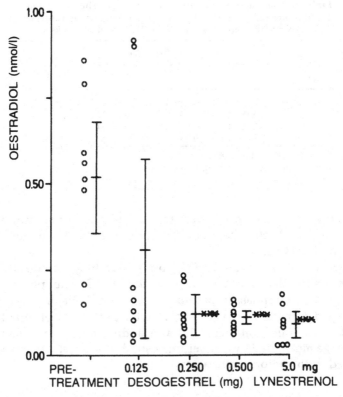

Figure 2 Individual serum levels of 17β-oestradiol in 8 fertile women before treatment on cycle day 7–9 and after 6 weeks of treatment with 5 mg lynestrenol, 0.125, 0.250 and 0.500 mg desogestrel. Treatments were given in a randomized order without intervals. Vertical bars represent means and ± 2 SEM. Statistical significances between pretreatment and treatment values are indicated with asterisks: * = $p < 1.25$, ** = $p < 0.01$ and *** = $p < 0.001$

SHBG levels were also significantly lowered during treatment (Figure 3). There was a highly significant correlation, with a correlation factor of 0.97, between SHBG and desogestrel dose except at the 0.125 mg level, while the SHBG – oestradiol correlation was weaker

($r = 0.54$). This indicates that oestradiol is not very efficient in regulating SHBG levels. This is borne out by the observation that postmenopausal and oophorectomized women have only slightly lower SHBG levels in spite of a lack of oestradiol in serum.

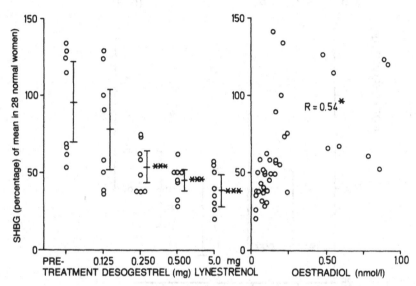

Figure 3 Left panel: Individual levels of S-SHBG determined by electroimmunoassay. Levels are given as percentages of a reference pool of serum from 28 untreated healthy fertile women. Volunteers, treatments and symbols as in Figure 2
Right panel: Correlation between SHBG and 17β-estradiol with pretreatment and treatment values given in Figures 2 and 4, left panel. R = correlation coefficient. * significant correlation, $p < 0.05$

It may be that the 19-nor-testosterone derivatives are blocking the SHBG-producing hepatocytes since the same has been found for levonorgestrel[6]. The 17α-hydroxyprogestogens, e.g. medroxyprogesteroneacetate, do not have this property. It is hardly an androgenic effect, since desogestrel *in vitro* has a low affinity to androgen receptors in comparison with levonorgestrel and testosterone[7]. As said in the introduction, desogestrel allows strong increases in SHBG by ethinyloestradiol in contrast to androgenic substances.

Desogestrel does not give any increase in prealbumin level (Figure

4). This is, however, seen with lynestrenol, indicating a weak androgenic rest effect in the latter.

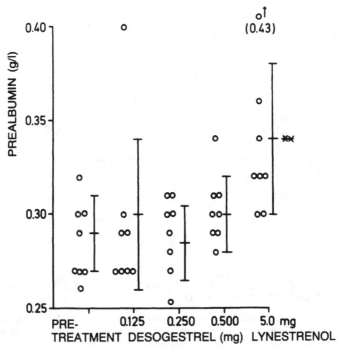

Figure 4 Individual levels of serum prealbumin in g/l. Volunteers, treatments and
symbols are the same as in Figure 2

In vaginal cytology another type of reaction is seen (Figure 5). Here,
despite adequate oestrogen levels in at least two cases, the maturation
value is depressed strongly, hinting at an antioestrogenic effect and
a lack of oestrogenic properties. The absence of an oestrogenic effect
can be inferred, since no changes in oestrogen-sensitive ceruloplasmin and CBG are found.

In conclusion, we found no signs of androgenic or oestrogenic
properties in desogestrel but a weak androgenic effect was detected

in lynestrenol. Evidence for antioestrogenic effect was found with both substances. Desogestrel is at least 10 times as potent as lynestrenol for the variables studied.

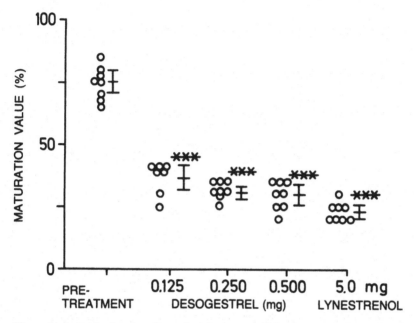

Figure 5 Individual maturation values in percent. Volunteers, treatments and symbols are the same as in Figure 2

References

1. Larsson-Cohn, U., Wallentin, L. and Zador, G. (1979). Plasma lipids and high density lipoproteins during oral contraception with different combinations of ethinylestradiol and levonorgestrel. *Horm. Metab. Res.*, **11**, 437
2. Miller, G. J. and Miller, N. E. (1975). Plasma-high-density-lipoprotein concentration and development of ischaemic heart disease. *Lancet*, **1**, 16
3. Cullberg, G., Dovre, P. A., Linstedt, G. and Steffensen, K. (1982). On the use of plasma proteins as indicators of the metabolic effects of combined oral contraceptives. *Acta Obstet. Gynecol. Scand. Suppl.*, **111**, 47
4. Laurell, C.-B. and Rannevik, G.-A. (1979). A comparison of plasma protein changes induced by danazol, pregnancy and oestrogens. *J. Clin. Endocrinol. Metab.*, **49**, 719
5. Barbosa, J., Seal, U. S. and Doe, R. P. (1971). Effects of anabolic steroids on hormone-binding proteins, serum cortisol and serum non-protein-bound cortisol. *J. Clin. Endocrinol.*, **32**, 232
6. Victor, A. and Johansson, E. D. B. (1977). Effects of d-norgestrel induced decreases in sex hormone binding globulin capacity on the d-norgestrel levels in plasma. *Contraception*, **16** (2), 115

7. Bergink, E. W., Hamburger, A. D., de Jager, E. and van der Vies, J. (1981). Binding of a contraceptive progestogen Org 2969 and its metabolites to receptor proteins and human sex hormone binding globulin. *J. Steroid Biochem.*, **14,** 175

3
Influence of a desogestrel/ ethinyloestradiol combination pill on sex hormone binding globulin and plasma androgens

E. KELLER, A. JASPER, M. ZWIRNER, H. UNTERBERG,
T. SCHUMACHER and A. E. SCHINDLER

SUMMARY

It is well known that (a) the progestogen desogestrel displays low affinity for androgen receptors and (b) that ethinyloestradiol stimulates the synthesis of sex hormone binding globulin (SHBG). Thus, it was the purpose of this study to evaluate the influence of a desogestrel/ethinyloestradiol combination pill on SHBG and plasma androgens.

During three cycles, eight female volunteers took a combination pill containing 0.15 mg desogestrel and 0.03 mg ethinyloestradiol daily for 21 days followed by a hormone-free interval of 7 days. Under the pill blood sampling was done weekly; in a control cycle before and after medication blood sampling was done every other day. The following parameters were determined: SHBG, testosterone (free and total), DHT, DHEA, DHEA sulphate, prolactin, oestradiol and progesterone.

Under the desogestrel/ethinyloestradiol combination a constant increase of SHBG could be observed which decreased again during the 7 days' hormone-free intervals but without reaching pretreatment levels. Plasma free testosterone and DHT revealed inverse patterns. One month after discontinuing the pill all parameters resumed pre-treatment values.

The results presented may explain the satisfactory situation concerning undesired androgenic effects under the desogestrel/ethinyl-oestradiol combination pill.

INTRODUCTION

In the female, low levels of sexual hormone binding globulin (SHBG) and high values of free testosterone are important factors for the manifestation of signs of androgenization such as acne and/or hirsutism[1]. While oestrogens stimulate SHBG synthesis and thus indirectly cause a decrease of free testosterone, androgens and also progestogens with androgenic rest activity lower SHBG levels. Consequently, in hormonal contraception the favourable oestrogen side-effect of SHBG stimulation can be neutralized according to the type and dose of the administered progestational substance. Obviously, this circumstance is of particular importance for the increasingly used low-dose oral contraceptives (i.e. oestrogen component < 0.04 mg)[2].

Since it is well known that the progestogen desogestrel – a potent progestational 19-nortestosterone derivative[3] – displays low affinity for androgen receptors[4], it was the purpose of this study to investigate the influence of a low-dose desogestrel/ethinyloestradiol combination pill on SHBG and plasma androgens.

MATERIALS AND METHODS

During three cycles, eight female volunteers (students; on average 24.6 years, 167 cm, 57 kg, menstrual cycles of 27–35 days; two smokers; seven practising oral contraception for the first time) took a combination pill containing 0.15 mg desogestrel and 0.03 mg ethinyloestradiol (Marvelon®) daily for 21 days followed by a 7-day hormonal-free interval. During treatment, venous blood sampling from a cubital vein was done once a week (days 1, 8, 15 and 22 of the cycle). In a control cycle before (control cycle 1) and after medication (control cycle 2) blood sampling was done every other day.

The following parameters were determined in serum or plasma: SHBG, free and total testosterone, dihydrotestosterone (DHT), dehydroepiandrosterone (DHEA), DHEA sulphate, LH, FSH, oestradiol, progesterone and prolactin.

The control cycles were centred around the day of the LH peak (indicated as day 0) as the day of presumed ovulation.

RESULTS

The control cycles before and after taking the desogestrel/ethinyloestradiol combination pill for 3 months did not reflect major differences: the duration of control cycle 1 was 32 days; the duration of control cycle 2 was 29 days (follicular phase: control cycle 1 = 20 days, control cycle 2 = 18 days; luteal phase: control cycle 1 = 12 days, control

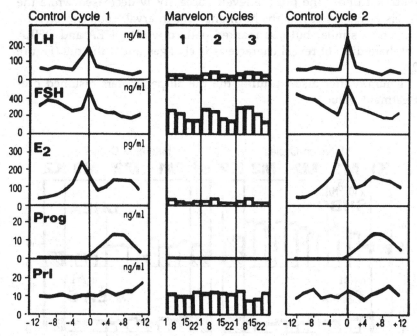

Figure 1   LH, FSH, oestradiol (E$_2$), progesterone (Prog), and prolactin (Prl) in a control cycle before treatment (Control Cycle 1), under three treatment cycles of a 0.15 mg desogestrel/0.03 mg ethinyloestradiol combination pill (Marvelon Cycles 1–3) and in a control cycle after treatment (Control Cycle 2); values are given as means

cycle 2 = 11 days). Both cycles revealed the classic criteria of ovulatory cycles: (1) perimenstrual FSH rise; (2) preovulatory oestradiol peak; (3) midcyclic LH and FSH peak; and (4) adequate progesterone secretion during the luteal phase (Figure 1).

27

During treatment with the pill there was a prompt suppression of LH, FSH, oestradiol and progesterone values, indicating a sufficient and reliable inhibition of ovulation already in the first treatment cycle.

In the course of all three treatment cycles a clear FSH rise after the 7-day hormonal-free interval could be observed (Figure 1).

Starting with the first treatment cycle there was a marked increase of SHBG by two-fold. During the 7-day hormonal-free interval a slight decrease of SHBG could be observed – but without reaching pretreatment values. Free testosterone and DHT revealed inverse patterns: under the pill the levels successively decreased while the levels increased during the hormonal-free interval. Total testosterone showed a similar but less marked pattern while DHEA and DHEA sulphate did not reveal characteristic changes under the pill (Figure 2).

1 month after discontinuing the pill all parameters resumed pre-treatment values.

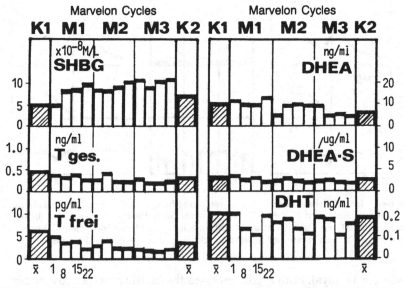

Figure 2 SHBG, total testosterone (T ges.), free testosterone (T frei), DHEA, DHEA sulphate and DHT in a control cycle before treatment (K1), under three treatment cycles of a 0.15 mg desogestrel/0.03 mg ethinyloestradiol combination pill (M1–M3), and in a control cycle after treatment (K2); values are given as means (x̄)

DISCUSSION

Already in the first treatment cycle of the desogestrel/ethinyloestra-diol combination pill a reliable inhibition of ovulation was noted by a sufficient suppression of the hypothalmic–pituitary–ovarian axis. Obviously, as in amenorrhoeic patients[5] FSH was the most insensitive parameter, followed by LH and oestradiol. After discontinuing the pill no change of corpus luteum quality could be observed in comparison with the pretreatment control cycle (Figure 1).

Significantly elevated SHBG levels and thus decreased free testosterone and DHT levels – which were reported after a 3 and 6 months treatment with the desogestrel/ethinyloestradiol combination pill[6,7] – could already be detected after the first 2 weeks of treatment. Although there was a slight decrease of SHBG during the 7 days' hormone free interval after having taken the pill for 21 days, SHBG levels remained elevated in comparison with pretreatment values so that the favourable effect of preventing undesired signs of androgenization is also available during the period of withdrawal bleeding.

Furthermore, the results presented may explain the fact that 73.2% of more than 1800 women with pre-existing acne reported an amelioration or a complete disappearance of acne having taken the desogestrel/ethinyloestradiol combination pill for more than 6 months[8].

References

1. Lawrence, D. M., Kate, M., Robinson, T. W. E., Newman, M. C., McGarrigle, H. H. C., Shaw, M. and Lachelin, G. C. L. (1981). Reduced sex hormone binding globulin and derived free testosterone levels in women with severe acne. *Clin. Endocrinol.*, **15**, 87
2. Taubert, H. D. and Kuhl, H. (1981). *Kontrazeption mit Hormonen.* (Stuttgart: Georg Thieme Verlag)
3. Visser de, F., de Jager, E., de Jongh, H. P., van der Vies, J. and Feellen, F. (1975). Pharmacological profile of a new orally active progestational compound. *Acta Endocrinol. (Copenh.)*, Suppl. **199**, 405
4. Bergink, E. W., Hamburger, A. D., de Jager, E. and van der Vies, J. (1981). Binding of a contraceptive progestogen Org 2969 and its metabolites to receptor proteins and human sex hormone binding globulin. *J. Steroid Biochem.*, **14**, 175
5. Keller, E. (1981). *Hypothalamus/Hypophysen – Funktiondiagnostik bei Amenorrhoe.* (Frankfurt: Peter D. Lang Verlag)
6. Bergink, E. W., Homa, P. and Pyörälä, T. (1983). Effects of oral contraceptive combination containing Levonorgestrel and Org 2969 on serum proteins and androgen binding. *Scand. J. Clin. Lab. Invest.* (In press)
7. Mall-Haefeli, M., Werner-Fodrow, J., Huber, P. and Weijers, M. J. (1982). Klinische

und biochemische Resultate bei der Behandlung mit Marvelon – einen neuen steroidalen Ovultationshemmer. *Gebuftsh. u. Frauenheilk.*, **42**, 215

8. Geissler, K-H. (1983). Hormonelle Kontrazeption mit Marvelon. *Fortschr. Med.*, **101**, 1060

4
Comparative haematological effects of new ethinyloestradiol–progestogen combinations

M. H. BRIGGS

SUMMARY

A randomized, prospective study on metabolic effects of three oral contraceptives is presented. The products used were a low-dose triphasic formulation of levonorgestrel (LNG) and ethinyloestradiol (EE), a fixed dose combination of 0.15 mg desogestrel (DOG) + 30 μg EE, and a sequential formulation of 50 μg EE ($\times$7), then 0.125 mg DOG + 50 μg EE ($\times$15). Over the initial six cycles significant changes were seen in coagulation and fibrinolytic factors in users of the sequential product, but much less with the other two products. Women using the sequential formulation were therefore switched to the triphasic product. After a further three cycles the laboratory tests showed restoration towards normality.

INTRODUCTION

Large epidemiological surveys of oral contraceptive (OC) users have suggested that some of the adverse clinical associations of OCs are related to the daily oestrogen dose, though others are related to the daily progestogen dose[1]. In an attempt to produce safer and more acceptable preparations, manufacturers have introduced a range of low-dose OC formulations. Particular attention has been placed on

31

the oestrogen component and most new formulations contain a daily dose of 30 or 35 μg ethinyloestradiol (EE). Recent evidence suggests that these low-oestrogen formulations have indeed reduced the incidence of some rare, but serious, side-effects of OCs[2,3]. A new progestogen (desogestrel (DOG), ORG 2969) has also been introduced and claimed to have a more favourable effect on laboratory indices of cardiovascular risk[4]. The present study was undertaken to compare the metabolic effects of three new OC formulations on young, healthy, new OC acceptors.

METHODS AND MATERIALS

The following commercial OC formulations were investigated: all contained EE combined with either levonorgestrel (LNG) or DOG.

(1) Triphasic: 0.050 mg LNG and 30 μg EE (×6); 0.075 mg LNG and 40 μg EE (×5); 0.125 mg LNG and 30 μg EE (×10).
(2) Monophasic: 0.150 mg DOG and 30 μg EE (×21).
(3) Biphasic: 50 μg EE (×7); 0.125 mg DOG and 50 μg EE (×15).

Criteria to enter the study included an absence of any absolute or relative contraindications to hormonal contraception, a body weight within 10% of the ideal for height, no concurrent medication, normotension, good personal motivation, age less than 30 years, and non-use of cigarettes. Written formal consent was obtained.

During the immediate pre-treatment cycle, all women used a barrier contraceptive: OCs were started on day 5 of the first treatment cycle.

Blood specimens were collected from the antecubital vein in subjects who had fasted overnight. Two specimens were taken on consecutive days during the late pre-treatment cycle (days 25–28) and during each treatment cycle on either of the last 2 days of pill taking.

Blood coagulation and fibrinolytic factors (fibrinogen, factor-VII, factor-VIII, factor-X, plasminogen, antithrombin-III) were measured every three cycles[5]. For logistic reasons, several laboratories collaborated in these measurements. All used the same quality control system.

RESULTS

At the time of preparing this report, 39 women had completed nine treatment cycles. Of these, 13 were receiving the monophasic product,

Table 1 Changes in coagulation and fibrinolytic factor activities. Results are given as percentages of pre-treatment values and are group means

	Cycle (treatment)								
	(150 μg DOG + 30 μg EE)			(Biphasic DOG + EE)			(Triphasic LNG + EE)		
Test	3	6	9	3	6	9†	3	6	9
Fibrinogen	110*	112*	113*	135***	146***	118**	108	110*	109
Coagulation factor:									
VII	108	110	111*	133***	140***	116**	104	105	103
VIII	106	107	110	121**	137***	112*	102	106	105
X	111*	113*	115*	135***	142***	115*	107	110*	108
Plasminogen	112*	116*	114*	142***	148***	116*	108	112*	110
Antithrombin-III	98	97	95	93***	88***	95	101	101	100

Difference between means significantly different: * $p < 0.5$; ** $p < 0.01$; *** $p < 0.001$.
†Subjects switched to triphasic treatment after cycle 6.

33

Table 2 Number of results outside normal reference ranges for coagulation and fibrinolytic factors

Factor	Cycle	150 μg DOG + 30 μg EE (n = 13)	Biphasic DOG + EE† (n = 14)	Triphasic LNG + EE (n = 12)
		Treatment		
Fibrinogen	0	0	0	0
	6	1	3	0
	9	2	2	0
Coagulation factor:				
VII	0	0	1	0
	6	1	4	1
	9	1	2	1
VIII	0	0	0	0
	6	2	3	0
	9	1	1	1
X	0	1	0	1
	6	1	4	0
	9	2	2	1
Plasminogen	0	0	1	1
	6	2	5	1
	9	1	2	1
AT-III	0	0	0	0
	6	1	4	1
	9	2	2	0
Total number of measurements of all factors		78	84	72
Total No. (%) of outliers	0	1 (1.3)	2 (2.4)	2 (2.8)
	6	8 (10.3)*	23 (27.4)***	3 (4.2)
	9	9 (11.5)*	11 (13.1)**	4 (5.6)

Difference between means significant: * $p < 0.05$; ** $p < 0.01$; *** $p < 0.001$.
†Subjects switched to triphasic treatment after cycle six.

34

14 the biphasic, and 12 the triphasic. As the changes in most factors in women using the biphasic were very large, it was decided for ethical reasons to transfer all of them to the triphasic product after six cycles. This should be borne in mind in interpreting the results (Table 1). In this table each woman served as her own control and results at three, six and nine cycles are expressed as a percentage of the pre-treatment cycle values.

Examination of individual values revealed a number to be outside the usual reference ranges. These are summarized in Table 2. Finally, as most women showed increases in levels of coagulation factors, but decreases in antithrombin-III, these changes can be emphasized by calculating the ratio of each factor to antithrombin-III (Table 3).

Table 3 Ratio of coagulation factors to antithrombin-III. Results are given as means and as percentages of mean values in cycle 0

	Cycle (treatment)					
	(150 μg DOG + 30 μg EE)		(Biphasic DOG + EE)		(Triphasic LNG+EE)	
	6	9	6	9†	6	9
Fibrinogen	115**	121**	166***	124**	109	109
Coagulation factor:						
VII	113*	116**	159***	122**	104	103
VIII	110	116**	156***	118**	105	105
X	116**	121**	161***	121**	109	108
Range	110–116	116–121	156–166	118–124	104–109	103–109
Mean	113*	119**	160***	121**	107	106

Difference between means significant: * $p < 0.05$; ** $p < 0.01$; *** $p < 0.001$.
†Subjects switched to triphasic treatment after cycle 6.

DISCUSSION AND CONCLUSIONS

Significant differences between the three products were apparent by cycles three and six, with large changes being seen in women using the biphasic formulation. While no cases of thrombosis were seen in any of the groups, it was considered prudent to transfer women on the biphasic to the triphasic product. As will be seen from the tables, by cycle nine there was a marked tendency for the abnormal results to become more normal, suggesting that the changes induced by the biphasic treatment are at least partially reversible by switching to a lower dose product.

While the two lower dose formulations produced much smaller changes in the various factors, fewer abnormalities were seen with the triphasic formulation containing LNG than with the monophasic product containing DOG.

On the basis of these findings, the biphasic formulation of DOG and EE does not seem suitable for routine use.

References

1. Royal College of General Practitioners (1974). *Oral Contraceptives and Health.* (London: Pitman)
2. Meade, T. W., Greenberg, G. and Thompson, S. C. (1980). Progestogens and cardiovascular reactions associated with oral contraceptives and a comparison of the safety of 50 and 30 μg oestrogen preparations. *Br. Med. J.*, **i**, 1157
3. Böttiger, L. E., Boman, G., Eklund, G. and Westerholm, B. (1980). Oral contraceptives and thromboembolic disease: effects of lowering oestrogen content. *Lancet*, **1**, 1097
4. Bergink, E. W., Hamburger, A. D., de Jager, E. and van der Vies, J. (1981). Binding of a contraceptive progestogen ORG 2969 and its metabolites to receptor proteins and human sex hormone binding globulin. *J. Steroid Biochem.*, **14**, 175
5. Triplett, D. A. and Harms, C. S. (1981). *Procedures for the Coagulation Laboratory.* (Chicago: American Society of Clinical Pathologists)

5
Oestroprogestogens and serum lipoproteins

F. R. HELLER and C. HARVENGT

SUMMARY

In the plasma, cholesterol (C) and triglycerides, are carried in five lipoprotein fractions: chylomicrons, very low density lipoproteins (VLDL), remnants, low density lipoproteins (LDL) and high density lipoproteins (HDL). Only remnants and LDL are implicated in the development of atherosclerosis; HDL, particularly HDL_2, are considered to be protective against atherosclerosis. Plasma VLDL and LDL are higher in the girls than in the boys. Women have less plasma total C and LDL-C and more plasma HDL-C than men. During the second part of the menstrual cycle, plasma levels of total C and LDL-C tend to be lower than in the first phase of the cycle. During pregnancy, plasma lipoproteins are elevated mainly during the third part of the pregnancy. In the postmenopausal period, women have a plasma lipoprotein pattern similar to that of men.

Both synthetic and natural oestrogens induced an increase in plasma VLDL and HDL (HDL_3) and a decrease in plasma LDL; these modifications could be considered as beneficial in terms of prevention of atherosclerosis. As far as the progestogens are concerned, the effects on plasma lipoproteins are opposed to those of oestrogens. The effects of the contraceptive pill on plasma lipoproteins will depend on the relative potency of its hormonal components, particularly of its progestogen component.

37

INTRODUCTION

After 20 years of oral contraceptive (OC) use, epidemiological data and scientific research have led to the now accepted evidence that the most important effect produced by these drugs on humans, other than the prevention of unwanted pregnancy, is an increase in the risk of cardiovascular disease. Because the incidence of cardiovascular disease is also related to disturbances of the lipoprotein metabolism, it appears to be opportune to analyse the different aspects of the interaction between female hormones and lipoprotein (LP) metabolism.

SERUM LIPOPROTEINS: METABOLISM

In the serum, lipids (cholesterol (C), triglycerides (TG), and phospholipids) are associated with peptides called apoproteins: apoproteins A-I, A-II, B, C, etc. The chylomicrons and the very low density lipoproteins (VLDL) are rich in TG and contain the Apo B-48; the low density lipoproteins (LDL) are rich in C and contain the Apo B-100; and the high density lipoproteins (HDL) are rich in proteins (Apo A-I, Apo A-II) and phospholipids.

The chylomicrons and the VLDL are secreted by the intestine and the liver and transformed into intermediary lipoproteins (IDL) called remnants; the LDL and the HDL can be considered as end products of the degradation of the TG-rich LP. The interconversion of some LP is regulated by lipolytic enzymes: lipoprotein lipase (LPL) which hydrolyses TG of the TG-rich LP; hepatic lipase (HL) which hydrolyses the phospholipids of the HDL; and the lecithin:cholesterol acyltransferase (LCAT) which esterifies C contained in the HDL_3 (the heaviest fraction of HDL) which are transformed in HDL_2; in this way, LCAT probably favours the transport of C toward the liver. Some LP, when in excess in the serum, such as remnants and LDL, are associated with a high risk of coronary heart disease; a rise in VLDL and chylomicronaemia can lead to pancreatitis and osteonecrosis. In contrast, high levels of HDL (HDL_2) could lower the risk of coronary heart disease.

FEMALE HORMONES AND CARDIOVASCULAR DISEASE

OCs have been found to increase the risk of venous thromboembolic diseases, particularly when no predisposing conditions are present. A direct correlation exists between the risk and the oestrogen content of OCs. The pathogenesis of thromboembolic disease caused by the OC appears to be related to the proliferation of various constituents of the vessel wall and to altered blood coagulation[1]. OCs also increase the risk of myocardial infarction, thrombotic stroke and haemorrhagic stroke[2].

Compared with non-users, the relative risk for myocardial infarction is increased for current users ($\times$3–4) and for long term (5 years or more) past users ($\times$2) for up to 10 years after drugs have been discontinued. Moreover, the risk is increased after the age of 40 and OCs multiply the effects of other risk factors (e.g. cigarette smoking, type II hyperlipoproteinaemia, diabetes mellitus). The pathogenesis of myocardial infarction attributable to OCs comprises two components: on one hand, an increase in the platelet hyperactivity and increased production and accumulation of fibrin; on the other hand, deleterious effects on blood pressure, glucose tolerance and HDL-C.

Recently, it has been suggested that the occurrence of all arterial diseases – ischaemic heart disease, cerebrovascular diseases, peripheral vascular disease and hypertension – can be directly related to the progestogen (19-nortestosterone derivative) dosage, which is itself inversely related to the serum HDL-C concentration[3]. Thus, it appears that arterial diseases could be linked to the use of female hormones through disturbances produced by these compounds on LP metabolism.

FEMALE HORMONES AND SERUM LIPOPROTEINS: PHYSIOLOGICAL STATES

The most dramatic changes in serum LP at the different periods of life of an individual occur during the first years of life and the levels approach those of young adults by 1–2 years of age; thereafter, the serum lipids levels remain relatively stable until the onset of puberty. During sexual maturation, a decline in serum TC, LDL-C, Apo B, HDL-C and Apo A-I is observed in both sexes but mainly in boys. This is followed by an increase during the late sexual development. In girls, HDL-C increase to the prepubertal concentration while in boys the level of HDL-C remains low. In contrast, serum TG show a continued increase with age in both sexes. After sexual maturation, females have higher serum concentrations of HDL (HDL_2), Apo A-I and Apo A-II and lower VLDL and IDL than males. So men exhibit progressively a more atherogenic LDL/HDL ratio with age but after menopause, levels of serum LP in females are somewhat similar to those in men[4,5].

During the menstrual cycle, serum TG rise to the highest concentration at mid-cycle and fall during the luteal phase; during the late luteal phase, there is a significant fall in plasma total C, LDL-C and Apo B but no change in the HDL-C and Apo A-I[6].

During pregnancy, serum TG and total C concentrations are elevated in 95% of women; TG-LP rises progressively and the serum TG exceed 2–3 times their basal level at the end of pregnancy, with a maximal rise in VLDL-TG. Total and VLDL-Apo B are also increased; LDL-Apo B has been found to be unchanged or elevated. After delivery, serum C and TG decrease but serum C can remain high until 6–7 weeks postpartum[7]. It is important to note that, at least in the human, LDL are the lipoproteins that are used by steroidogenic tissues such as the adrenal cortex and the ovarian corpus luteum as a source of hormones.

FEMALE HORMONES AS A CAUSE OF DISORDERS IN LIPOPROTEIN METABOLISM

OCs have been shown to increase serum TG and total C concentration. Population studies from the Lipid Research Clinics Programme indicated that serum TG levels were approximately 50% higher and total-C 5–7% higher in young users of oral contraceptives, while in women aged 55 years and over, using hormone preparations (presumably oestrogens), there was a modest decline in mean cholesterol of about 5–6% and a slight but variable increase (maximum 5%) in triglycerides in comparison with non-users. Several studies have suggested that the alterations in serum levels of the different LP are related to the oestrogen/progestin potency of the contraceptive pill[8]. This was emphasized in a recent report from the Lipid Research Clinics Prevalence Study[9]. It appears that LDL-C concentrations are highest in women using low-dose oestrogen oral contraceptives (14–24%) and indistinguishable from the levels in non-users when high dose oestrogen oral contraceptives with strong progestin potency (taking into account the type and dosage) are used. With equine oestrogens, the LDL-C levels are 12% higher in younger women and 11–19% lower in postmenopausal women than in non-users.

On the other hand, the levels of HDL-C are significantly higher than in non-users and tend to be highest in users of oestrogen-dominant preparations and lowest in users of progestin-dominant preparations.

It must be remembered that the androgenic progestogens of the 19-nortestosterone (levonorgestrel) series reverse the beneficial effect of postmenopausal oestrogen treatment on HDL-C whereas among the hydroxyprogesterone derivatives, medroxyprogesterone acetate has no such effect[10]. Desogestrel, although displaying stronger progestational activity than levonorgestrel seems to produce *in vivo* effects similar to those of levonorgestrel on serum lipoproteins at the same dosage. The increase in the HDL-C observed with some contraceptive pills is accounted for primarily by an increase in HDL_3 mass in contrast with the findings in postmenopausal users of natural oestrogens, in whom increased levels of HDL are confined to the HDL_2 species[11]. On the other hand, norgestrel has been reported to lower HDL_2 concentrations.

Whole serum and LDL, HDL and VLDL triglycerides concentrations are significantly elevated in both older and younger women using sex hormones[9]. The analysis of the data clearly shows that the oestrogenic component of oral contraceptives is associated with higher TG levels[8], and that certain progestins oppose the action of the oestrogens and lower TG levels. That the changes in HDL-C and TG during oral contraceptive treatment are influenced by the total oestrogenicity of the drug is also suggested by the positive correlation found between the mean changes in HDL-C or TG levels and the mean changes in the plasma concentration of sex hormone binding globulin and with the ethinyloestradiol–levonorgestrel ratio[12].

Finally, the cholesterol content of the VLDL is elevated in women using contraceptive pills[9]; this finding may signify increased serum concentration of remnants that are associated with accelerated atherosclerosis. The low-dose triphasic contraceptive pills seem to induce little changes in the serum lipid fractions. However, recent data show that it can be misleading because the serum Apo-B levels have been found to be significantly increased by a triphasic contraceptive pill, although the changes in lipid fractions have been very small and the ratio LDL-C/HDL-C unaltered[13]. High serum Apo-B level is

41

correlated to an increased risk of coronary heart disease. Preliminary studies have shown that the combination of desogestrel with ethinyl-oestradiol could have beneficial (increase of HDL-C and Apo A-I) or less detrimental effects (lower increase of VLDL, absence or increase of Apo B) on the serum lipoprotein pattern than other combinations[14,15], but these results have not been uniformly confirmed and more studies are needed with this compound.

In order to avoid high peaks of serum hormone concentrations and the hepatic first pass, natural oestrogens have been administered by a non-oral route. Percutaneous administration of oestradiol does not seem to alter the lipoprotein pattern[16]; with the hormone releasing vaginal rings, the LDL-C/HDL-C ratio tends to be higher when ethinyloestradiol is combined with levonorgestrel and unmodified when oestradiol is combined with the progesterone-derivatives progestins[17].

The occurrence of pregnancy and oestrogen therapy can lead to massive hypertriglyceridaemia (levels above $2000 \, \text{mg} \, \text{dl}^{-1}$) with chylomicronaemia in women suffering from familial hypertriglyceridaemia but curiously not from familial combined hyperlipoproteinaemia or dysbetalipoproteinaemia.

FEMALE HORMONES AS A TREATMENT OF DISORDERS IN LIPOPROTEIN METABOLISM

In dysbetalipoproteinaemia, in fact, lower TG levels can be observed with oestrogen treatment[18]; this paradoxal effect of oestrogens could be related to an accelerated catabolism of remnants by the liver. Another beneficial effect of oestrogens may be the type II hyperlipoproteinaemia encountered in postmenopausal women[19]. Finally, two 19-nortestosterone derivatives, oxandrolone (an anabolic steroid) and norethindrone acetate (a progestogen), have been shown to reduce the plasma and VLDL-TG in various hyperlipoproteinaemias[20]. It must be remembered that oestrogens have been found to increase the risk of myocardial infarction in men (Coronary Drug Project), but to lower the same risk in post-menopausal women[21].

FEMALE HORMONES AND REGULATION OF LIPID METABOLISM

Plasma LPL activity is lower in women before puberty and becomes similar to or higher than men after puberty; plasma LH activity is lower in women after puberty although sometimes no sex-linked differences are seen in LPL and LH. During the luteal phase of the menstrual cycle, the plasma LPL activator property is increased[22]. During pregnancy, high adipose tissue LPL may facilitate increased TG uptake and fat deposition in adipose tissue; at the end of pregnancy and during lactation, the mammary tissue LPL is increased perhaps to shunt circulating TG from adipose depots to mammary tissue for milk synthesis[23]. The changes in LPL activity in these tissues seem to be related to prolactin secretion. The plasma LCAT activity is higher in males than females but the LCAT mass estimated by a radioimmunoassay (RIA) tend to be lower in males than females. Evaluated by RIA, the LCAT is similar in women with and without oestrogen replacement or oral contraceptives[24].

Rats treated with oestrogens exhibit low rates of ketogenesis and high rates of TG secretion and the hypertriglyceridaemia induced by oestrogen has been usually related to the increased TG products by the liver[25]; moreover, in roosters the Apo-B synthesis is stimulated by oestrogens. However, a decrease in plasma post-heparin lipolytic activity has been demonstrated for oestrogens and OCs, presumably due to a selective suppression in HL[26]. In men with prostatic carcinoma, the plasma LCAT activity is increased by oestrogens and cyproterone acetate, while in rats, progestogens inhibit plasma LCAT activity *in vitro* but not *in vivo*. Progestins of the 19-nortestosterone derivatives but not of the medroxyprogesterone derivatives induce an increase of HL which is significantly correlated with the decrease in plasma HDL_2[27].

The use of OCs is associated with a significant increase in biliary C saturation caused by an increase in C secretion and a decrease in bile acid secretion[28]. The saturation of bile with C is found also during the luteal phase and during the second and third trimester of pregnancy.

In rats, pharmacological doses of 17α-ethinyloestradiol cause a profound lowering of plasma C and LP by increasing the number of hepatic receptors for human LDL (Apo B), and so the rate of catabolism of LP[29]. On the other hand, in rabbits, oestrogen increases hepatic uptake of VLDL and LDL which are rich in Apo E[30].

Serum lipoproteins are modified quantitatively and qualitatively by sex and sex hormones, depending on the relative oestrogen/progestin potency. These changes could be or seem to be different whether the hormones are given as natural or synthetic compounds, whether the oral or the non-oral route is used, and sometimes are influenced by the pre-existing lipoprotein status and the menopause. In terms of atherosclerosis, evaluation of the effects of female hormones on serum lipoproteins must take into account not only the lipid content (HDL-C, LDL-C), but perhaps more importantly the peptide components of these lipoproteins (Apo A-I, Apo B). The hormonal contraception to be selected by the clinician must be proved not to impair the lipoprotein metabolism and special caution has to be taken before prescribing progestin-dominant oral contraceptives; presently, the ideal combination has still to be found.

References

1. Stadel, B. V. (1981). Oral contraceptives and cardiovascular disease (part I). *N. Engl. J. Med.*, **305,** 612
2. Stadel, B. V. (1981). Oral contraceptives and cardiovascular disease (part II). *N. Engl. J. Med.*, **305,** 672
3. Wingrave, S. J. (1982). Progestogen effects and their relationship of lipoprotein changes. *Acta Obstet. Gynecol. Scand.*, **105,** (Suppl.), 33
4. Connor, S. L., Connor, W. E., Sexton, G., Calvin, L. and Bacon, S. (1982). The effects of age, body weight and family relationships on plasma lipoprotein and lipids in men, women and children of randomly selected families. *Circulation*, **65,** 1290
5. Riesen, W. F., Mordasini, R. C. and Oetliker, O. H. (1983). Les altérations de la composition des lipoproteins sériques durant l'ontogénèse. In Van Keep, P. A. and de Gennes, J. L. (eds.). *Contraceptifs Oraux et Lipoproteines*, pp. 34–41. (Paris: Masson)
6. Kim, H. J. and Kalkhoff, R. K. (1979). Changes in lipoprotein composition during the menstrual cycle. *Metabolism*, **28,** 663
7. Hillman, L., Schonfeld, G., Miller, J. P. and Wulff, G. (1975). Apolipoproteins in human pregnancy. *Metabolism*, **24,** 943
8. Bradley, D. D., Wingerd, J., Petitti, D., Krauss, R. M. and Ramcharan, S. (1978). Serum high-density-lipoprotein cholesterol in women using oral contraceptives, estrogens and progestins. *N. Engl. J. Med.*, **299,** 17
9. Wahl, P., Walden, C., Knopp, R., Hoover, J., Wallace, R., Heiss, G. and Rifkind, B. (1983). Effect of estrogen/progestin potency on lipid/lipoprotein cholesterol. *N. Engl. J. Med.*, **308,** 862
10. Hirvonen, E., Mälkönen, M. and Manninen, V. (1981). Effects of different progestogens on lipoproteins during postmenopausal replacement therapy. *N. Engl. J. Med.*, **304,** 560
11. Krauss, R. M., Roy, S., Mishell, D. R., Jr., Casagrande, J. and Pike, M. C. (1983). Effects of two low-dose oral contraceptives on serum lipids and lipoproteins: Differential changes in high-density lipoprotein subclasses. *Am. J. Obstet. Gynecol.*, **145,** 446

TRENDS IN ORAL CONTRACEPTION

12. Larsson-Cohn, U., Fahraeus, L., Wallentin, L. and Zador, G. (1981). Lipoprotein changes may be minimized by proper composition of a combined oral contraceptive. *Fertil. Steril.*, **35**, 172
13. Harvengt, C., Desager, J. P. and Lecart, C. (1983). Effects of plasma apoproteins A-I and B induced by two estrogestin preparations: monophasic versus triphasic. *Curr. Ther. Res.*, **33**, 385
14. Samsioe, G. (1982). Comparative effects of the oral contraceptive combinations 0.150 mg desogestrel + 0.030 mg ethinyloestradiol and 0.150 mg levonorgestrel + 0.030 mg ethinyloestradiol on lipid and lipoprotein metabolism in healthy female volunteers. *Contraception*, **25**, 487
15. De Jager, E. and Bergink, E. W. (1981). New progestagens for oral contraception. In Van der Molen, H. J., Klopper, A., Lunenfeld B., *et al.* (eds.). *Hormonal Factors in Fertility and Contraception. Research on Steroids*, Vol. **10**, pp. 122–31. (Amsterdam: Excerpta Medica)
16. Basdevant, A. and Guy-Grand, B. (1983). Influence de la voie d'administration sur les effets hormonaux et métaboliques de l'oestrogenotherapie. In Van Keep, P. A. and de Gennes, J. L. (eds.). *Contraceptifs Oraux et Lipoproteins*, pp. 85–9. (Paris: Masson)
17. Lithell, H., Ahren, T., Odlind, V., Weiner, E., Vessby, B., Victor, A. and Johnsson, E. D. B. (1983). Effects of progestins on lipoprotein patterns. In Bartin, C. W., Milgröm, E. and Mauvais-Jarvis, P. (eds.). *Progesterone and Progestins*, pp. 421–32. (New York: Raven Press)
18. Kushwaha, R. S., Hazzard, W. R., Gagne, C., Chait, A. and Albers, J. J. (1977). Type III hyperlipoproteinemia: paradoxical hypolipidemic response to estrogen. *Ann. Intern. Med.*, **87**, 515
19. Tikkanen, M., Nikkila, E. A. and Vartiainen, E. (1978). Natural oestrogen as an effective treatment for type-II hyperlipoproteinaemia in postmenopausal women. *Lancet*, **2**, 490
20. Tamai, T., Nakai, T., Yamada, S., *et al.* (1979). Effects of oxandrolone on plasma lipoproteins in patients with type IIa, IIb and IV hyperlipoproteinemia: occurrence of hypo-high density lipoproteinemia. *Artery*, **5**, 125
21. Bain, C., Willett, W., Hennekens, C. H., Rosner, B., Belangers, C. and Speizer, F. E. (1981). Use of postmenopausal hormones and risk of myocardial infarction. *Circulation*, **64**, 42
22. de Mendoza, S. G., Nucete, H., Salazar, E., Zerpa, A. and Kashyap, M. L. (1979). Plasma lipids and lipoprotein lipase activator property during the menstrual cycle. *Horm. Metab. Res.*, **11**, 696
23. Steingrimsdottir, L., Brasel, J. A. and Greenwood, M. R. C. (1980). Diet, pregnancy, and lactation: Effects on adipose tissue, lipoprotein lipase, and fat cell size. *Metabolism*, **29**, 837
24. Albert, J. J., Bergelin, R. O., Adolphson, J. L. and Wahl, P. W. (1982). Population-based reference values for lecithin-cholesterol acyltransferase (LCAT). *Atherosclerosis*, **43**, 369
25. Glueck, C. J., Fallat, R. W. and Scheel, D. (1975). Effects of estrogenic compounds on triglyceride kinetics. *Metabolism*, **24**, 537
26. Applebaum, D. M., Goldberg, P., Pykälistö, O. J., Brunzell, J. D. and Hazzard, W. R. (1977). Effect of estrogen on post-heparin lipolytic activity. Selective decline in hepatic triglyceride lipase. *J. Clin. Invest.*, **59**, 601
27. Nikkilä, E. A., Tikkanen, M. J. and Kuusi, T. (1983). Effects of progestins on plasma lipoproteins and heparin-releasable lipases. In Bartin, C. W., Milgröm, E. and Mauvais-Jarvis, P. (eds.). *Progesterone and Progestins*, pp. 411–20. (New York: Raven Press)
28. Kern, F., Jr., Everson, G. T., De Mark, B., McKinley, C., Showalter, R. and

Braverman, D. Z. (1982). Biliary lipids, bile acids and gallbladder function in the human female: effects of contraceptive steroids. *J. Lab. Clin. Med.*, **99**, 798

29. Kovanen, P. T., Brown, M. S. and Goldstein, J. L. (1979). Increased binding of low density lipoprotein to liver membranes from rats treated with 17α-ethinyl estradiol. *J. Biol. Chem.*, **254**, 11367

30. Floren, C. H., Kushwaha, R. S., Hazzard, W. R. and Albers, J. J. (1981). Estrogen-induced increase in uptake of cholesterol-rich very low density lipoproteins in perfused rabbit liver. *Metabolism*, **30**, 367

6
Cycle control and modern contraception: some relevant aspects

M. J. WEIJERS

SUMMARY

Literature data regarding cycle control of oral contraceptives are often unclear because of the lack of information on definitions concerning the evaluation of clinical trials. This frequently makes a valid comparison of results from different studies impossible. Information considered to be meaningful for practical purposes is discussed. Based on experience from multicentre trials with 14 000 women involving 180 000 cycles with combinations containing varying doses of a progestational and an oestrogenic substance, details are given about the role these active substances play in cycle control.

It is demonstrated that the progestational and oestrogenic components have independent influences on spotting and breakthrough bleeding. Predictions regarding cycle control, based only on the ratio progestogen to oestrogen, should not be made.

Since the introduction of oral contraceptives (OCs) in the late 1950s, the main issues with these preparations have been reliability, cycle control and safety. In comparison with other methods of contraception, OCs have an outstanding reliability[1]. Although the reliability of OCs can be assessed by various methods of calculation, the data obtained should reflect as close as possible the situation as it occurs in daily clinical practice. A relevant question raised in this context is whether pregnancies due to improper use of OCs should be included in the reporting. As appears from literature data, in daily practice up to 8% of women using OCs forget to take a tablet each day[2]. In addition it is known that the reliability of OCs may become impaired as a consequence of drug–OC interactions[3]. The implications of these aspects are growing in view of the continuing dose reductions of both the progestogen and oestrogen component of low-dose OCs[3]. This seems to be particularly valid in the case of the so-called triphasics, where dose reduction apparently has reached a critical point and, as a result, contraceptive failures begin to occur[4-7].

As far as safety is concerned, today there is a fair deal of understanding about the risks and benefits of OCs. With respect to the undesirable effects, attention has been focussed on the cardiovascular hazards, a topic that has been dealt with extensively in numerous epidemiological and biochemical studies[8,9]. Later, when the studies continued, it appeared that the risks had been overstated and were actually very small[10]. In addition it has become clear that future investigations should concentrate on the underlying mechanisms in order to identify those women who are at greater risk of developing serious adverse effects[11]. In contrast to the health risks, the health benefits of OCs have been almost ignored during the past 20 years of their use. However, fortunately times are changing and evidence is accumulating that the benefits of OC use far outweigh the risks[12].

Although there exists a vast bibliography on OCs, relatively little attention has been paid to control of bleeding, since scientifically reliable studies on cycle control are scarce. There is little meaning in presenting data on the incidence of spotting, breakthrough bleeding (BTB) and missing periods if information on the general design of the study, on the definitions of bleeding parameters and on the population concerned is inadequate or lacking. In addition, most reports have failed to provide detailed information on the various groups of women studied, for example on switchers or new starters and on the age distribution of the women. Besides, information on compliance with regular tablet intake and on the reasons for discontinuing OC treatment (drop-outs) is rare. There is also little meaning in presenting data on control of bleeding that have been 'corrected' for pre-treatment cycle irregularities[13], since this has no affinity with daily OC practice.

It needs no argument that this inadequacy of information does not present the physician with much opportunity to make a so-called 'educated selection of an oral contraceptive'[14]. To what amazing results the above-mentioned omissions and inconsistencies in reporting may lead can be illustrated best by looking at the following literature data.

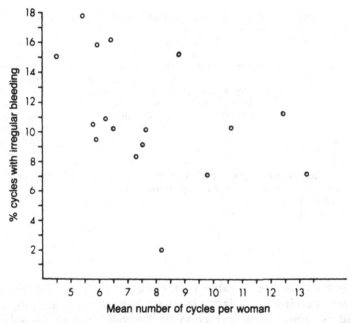

Figure 1 Mean incidence of irregular bleeding (breakthrough bleeding and spotting) as obtained with an oral contraceptive containing 0.15 mg levonorgestrel and 0.03 mg ethinyloestradiol in 16 different investigations. Reproduced by kind permission from reference 15

With a low-dose OC, containing 0.03 mg ethinyloestradiol (EE) and 0.15 mg levonorgestrel data on bleeding irregularities have been reported which were obtained in 16 different investigations[15]. Figure 1 shows the mean number of cycles with irregular bleeding (IB; calculated as a percentage over the total number of cycles per trial), in relation to the mean number of cycles per woman obtained in each trial. As can be seen the mean incidence of IB varied widely in these trials, ranging from 2 to 18%. Although cycle control may differ between different ethnic groups, it is unlikely that the wide variation in IB can be explained merely by this aspect.

In another paper, cycle control data on a so-called 'triphasic' preparation were produced referring only to the women who did not forget to take any tablet and to the women with a history of no

Table 1 The incidence of irregular bleeding with a triphasic preparation*

	Trial A (6628 cycles)[†]		Trial B (25 000 cycles)		
	All cycles, excluding women who forgot tablets	All cycles, excluding women with irregular bleeding in anamnesis	cycles[‡] 1	6	12
% cycles with irregular bleeding	7.8	6.5	23.8	16.0	11.5

*6 × 0.03 mg ethinyloestradiol (EE) + 0.05 mg levonorgestrel; 5 × 0.04 mg EE + 0.075 mg levonorgestrel; 10 × 0.03 mg EE + 0.125 mg levonorgestrel.
[†]From reference 13.
[‡]Without corrections. From reference 16.

bleeding irregularities[13]. Table 1 compares these 'corrected' figures with those obtained in a fairly large study by another investigator who did not apply such 'corrections'[16]. It should be noted that both studies are comparable for the mean number of treatment cycles per woman.

In view of these discrepancies, the relevance for clinical practice of presenting corrected data should be questioned seriously! In addition, it will be clear from the above that comparisons of various data on cycle control published so far will contribute neither to a better understanding nor facilitate a proper evaluation and/or selection of an OC.

It has been suggested that spotting and BTB are influenced not only by the amount of oestrogen in an OC but also by the ratio of the amount of oestrogen and progestogen[17]. Although over the years many cycle control data have been produced with a variety of high- and low-dose OCs, there is still poor understanding about the influence of the oestrogen/progestogen component of an OC on bleeding parameters.

Since March 1976 our group has collected a large number of data on cycle control, obtained in various multicentre clinical trials with 19 different experimental desogestrel/EE combinations. The studies covered 14 000 women who were treated during 180 000 cycles. Because throughout these studies the same definitions (including those for control of bleeding) were used, the data obtained can be compared and consequently the influence of the oestrogen and progestogen components on cycle control can be examined.

The following definitions for control of bleeding were applied:

(1) Spotting: a scanty bleeding, starting outside the tablet-free period, which does not require any hygienic measures or at most one sanitary towel per day.

(2) BTB: bleeding, starting outside the tablet-free period, which is not a spotting and which cannot be considered as a withdrawal bleeding.

(3) Withdrawal bleeding: a bleeding that begins in the tablet-free period.

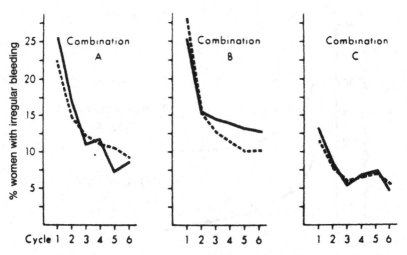

Figure 2 The influence of extension of the trial on irregular bleeding with three oral contraceptive combinations. Combination A: — = 530 women in cycle 1, 234 in cycle 6; — — — = 1609 in cycle 1, 1244 in cycle 6. Combination B: — = 419 women in cycle 1, 298 in cycle 6; — — — = 1044 in cycle 1, 837 in cycle 6. Combination C: — = 351 women in cycle 1, 256 in cycle 6; — — — = 686 in cycle 1, 589 in cycle 6

51

In addition, it should be emphasized that in every study the percentage of switchers and new starters was kept fairly constant (45–55% for each group) and that at least 10 centres were involved.

A basic question with respect to cycle control with an OC refers to the number of data needed to obtain a fairly accurate idea about the incidence of IB. This aspect is illustrated in Figure 2 for three different OC combinations. As can be seen, extension of the trial beyond 200 women per cycle hardly influences the incidence of IB. Figure 2 also shows that with all combinations the incidence of IB is higher during the first 1–3 treatment cycles, while it stabilizes soon at much lower levels on continuation of treatment. It needs no argument in this context that for a proper judgment of an OC the prescribing physician needs a specification of the incidence of IB per cycle.

As stated above, the role of the oestrogen and progestogen components in control of bleeding is far from clear. In Figure 3 two desogestrel/EE combinations are compared that have the same progestogen:oestrogen ratio. Figure 3 shows that this ratio is not the only factor that determines the incidence of IB. Apparently, as already

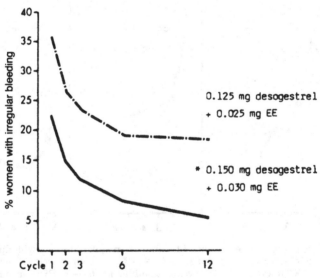

Figure 3 The influence of progestogen:oestrogen ratio on the incidence of irregular bleeding. EE = Ethinyloestradiol; *Marvelon

suggested[17], the amounts of oestrogen and/or progestogen also contribute to the ultimate effect. This is illustrated in Figures 4 and 5.

By comparing three OC combinations (Figure 4), each containing the same amount of EE (0.05 mg) but an increasing amount of desogestrel, the influence of the progestogen dose on the incidence of BTB

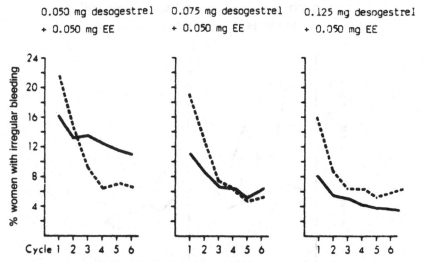

Figure 4 The influence of increasing progestogen dose on the incidence of irregular bleeding with oral contraceptive combinations containing 0.05 mg ethinyloestradiol (EE). — = Breakthrough bleeding; — — — = spotting

and spotting could be examined. As can be seen from Figure 4, the incidence of BTB decreases when the progestogen dose increases. The consistency of this phenomenon has been demonstrated also in the case of combinations that contain a dose of 0.03 mg EE and an increasing amount of desogestrel. This strongly suggests that it is primarily the amount of progestogen in an OC that influences the occurrence of BTB.

53

On the other hand, it appears that the oestrogen dose is the major determining factor for spotting. This is very well illustrated by Figure 5, which shows that in the presence of the same dose of desogestrel, spotting substantially decreases when the oestrogen dose is increased from 0.03 mg EE to 0.05 mg EE.

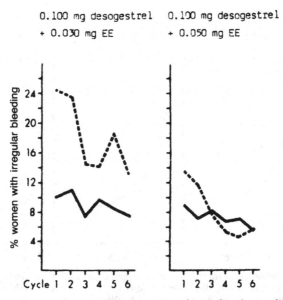

Figure 5 The influence of an increasing oestrogen dose (ethinyloestradiol, EE) on the incidence of irregular bleeding with oral contraceptive combinations containing 0.1 mg desogestrel. — = Breakthrough bleeding; — — — = spotting

Summarizing with respect to control of bleeding the following conclusions can be made:

(1) Reports should contain all definitions applied to the study.
(2) No corrections should be made for events that are known to

exist during the daily use of OCs, such as forgetting tablets and a history of irregular bleeding.

(3) For adequate assessment of cycle control with an OC, the data should refer to at least 200 women, treated during six cycles, and should be obtained in at least 10 centres. Extension of a trial from 200 to 600 or more women per cycle changes the mean incidence of IB only by 2–3%.

(4) The oestrogen and progestogen components of OCs each play a separate role in the occurrence of BTB and spotting. No indication was found for a so-called 'optimal oestrogen/progestogen-dose relationship'.

References

1. Vessey, M. (1982). Efficacy of different contraceptive methods. *Lancet*, **1**, 841
2. N.I.S.S.O. (Nederlands Instituut voor Sociaal Sexuologisch Onderzoek) (1975). *Anticonceptiegedrag. Verslag van een onderzoek bij 1200 nederlandse vrouwen en mannen naar de wijze waarop men een zwangerschap probeert te voorkomen.* (Report on an investigation in 1200 Dutch women and men with respect to their ways of preventing pregnancy). (Zeist: N.I.S.S.O.)
3. Orme, M. L. E. (1982). The clinical pharmacology of oral contraceptive steroids. *Br. J. Clin. Pharmacol.*, **14**, 31
4. Fay, R. A. (1982). Failure with the new triphasic oral contraceptive Logynon. *Br. Med. J.*, **284**, 17
5. Graham, H. (1982). Failure with the new triphasic oral contraceptive Logynon. *Br. Med. J.*, **284**, 422
6. Cullberg, G., et al. (1982). Two oral contraceptives, efficacy, serum proteins, and lipid metabolism. *Contraception*, **26**, 229
7. Cullberg, G. (1983). Säkerheten hos lagdoserade p-piller-metodfel en biverkning? (Reliability of low-dose contraceptive pill-method error a side effect?) *Läkartidningen*, **80**, 2484
8. Johns Hopkins University (1982). *Population Reports. Oral Contraceptives in the 1980s*, Series A, No. 6, A189–A221. (Baltimore: Johns Hopkins University)
9. Briggs, M. H. and Briggs, M. (1981). Metabolic effects of oral contraceptives. In Fen, C. C., et al. (eds.). *Recent Advances in Fertility Regulation*. Proceedings of a symposium on recent advances in fertility regulation. Beijing 2–5 September 1980, pp. 83–111. (Geneva: S. A. Atar)
10. Wiseman, R. A. and MacRae, K. D. (1981). Oral contraceptives and the decline in mortality from circulatory disease. *Fertil. Steril.*, **35**, 277
11. Kay, C. R. (1980). The happiness pill? *J. R. Coll. Gen. Pract.*, **30**, 8
12. Mishell, D. R. (1982). Noncontraceptive health benefits of oral steroidal contraceptives. *Am. J. Obstet. Gynecol.*, **142**, 809
13. Lachnit-Fixson, U. (1979). Erstes Dreistufenpraeparat zur hormonalen Konzeptionsverhuetung, Klinische Ergebnisse. *Muench. Med. Wochenschr.*, **121**, 1421
14. Woutersz, T. B. (1981). A low-dose combination oral contraceptive. *J. Reprod. Med.*, **26**, 615
15. Bergstein, N. A. M. (1976). Clinical efficacy, acceptability and metabolic effects of new low dose combined oral contraceptives. *Acta Obstet. Gynecol. Scand. Suppl.*, **54**, 51

16. Upton, G. V. (1982). Clinical experience with triphasics. Presented at the *San Francisco Congress, October 17–22*
17. Lawson, J. S. (1979). Optimum dosage of an oral contraceptive. *Am. J. Obstet. Gynecol.*, **134**, 315

7
Studies with desogestrel for fertility regulation

J. R. NEWTON

INTRODUCTION

Over the past 20 years Organon have been involved in developing a new series of progestogens characterized by the absence of an oxygen at position 3 of the steroid skeleton. Following lynestrenol, the most promising compound in early trials was desogestrel, a 13-ethyl-11-methylene-3-desoxy compound, which is a more specific progestogen than both norethisterone and levonorgestrel[1]. Receptor binding studies have demonstrated a lower affinity of the main metabolite of desogestrel for androgen receptors than levonorgestrel[1].

A large multicentre trial indicated that a combination of $150 \mu g$ desogestrel and $30 \mu g$ ethinyloestradiol (Marvelon) was an effective oral contraceptive (pregnancy rate $0.1 (\text{woman-year})^{-1}$) and caused a low level of irregular bleeding and side-effects[2]. Further work has suggested that this combination elevates HDL-cholesterol levels compared with a combination of $150 \mu g$ levonorgestrel and $30 \mu g$ oestradiol (Microgynon)[3,4].

In January 1982, prior to its introduction in the UK, a limited acceptability trial of Marvelon was initiated. The aim was to investigate the efficacy and tolerance of this new pill in the British family planning clinic population.

Recently considerable interest has been directed towards the effect of different hormonal contraceptive formulations on HDL cholesterol.

Epidemiological studies have demonstrated an inverse relationship between this parameter and ischaemic heart disease[5]. For this reason a randomized comparative study of Marvelon and Microgynon was conducted on a sub-group of patients participating in the acceptability trial.

PATIENTS AND METHODS

Twelve family planning clinics participated in the acceptability trial and recruited 238 suitable patients within a 3-month period.

In four centres 70 of these patients were randomly allocated to either Marvelon or Microgynon only for comparison of the effects on serum lipoproteins and SHBG.

Patients selected were healthy, of fertile age, having a regular cycle and with risk of pregnancy. No patient who had employed any hormonal preparation within 3 months was included. Other exclusion criteria were those standard contraindications to oral contraceptives, including breast-feeding women and those receiving any drug with a known interaction with oral contraceptives. Informed consent was obtained before treatment.

Marvelon tablets containing $150\,\mu g$ desogestrel and $30\,\mu g$ ethinyloestradiol were taken daily for 21 days, commencing on the first day of menstrual bleeding. There was a 7-day treatment-free interval before the next treatment cycle and each patient was assessed over six treatment cycles. Microgynon was administered in an identical manner.

After selection for the trial a brief gynaecological history was taken and a physical examination, which included measurement of blood pressure and weight, was performed.

Follow-up visits were after one, three and six cycles, at which blood pressure, weight and side-effects were recorded. Patients were required to complete diary cards for recording bleeding patterns and tablet compliance and these were collected at each clinic visit.

The following definitions were used:

(1) Withdrawal bleeding: bleeding beginning during the tablet-free period (days 22–28).

(2) Spotting: scanty bleeding occurring during tablet intake, requiring a minimum of sanitary protection.

(3) Breakthrough bleeding: bleeding occurring during tablet intake, requiring two or more sanitary pads per day.

The patients who agreed to participate in the serum lipoprotein study also provided a fasting (12 hour) blood sample before treatment and after three and six cycles. Wherever possible, during treatment blood samples were collected in the third week of each cycle.

After centrifugation serum was collected and stored at $-20°$C until analysis for total cholesterol, HDL cholesterol, triglycerides and SHBG. All serum protein and lipid analysis was performed in one laboratory and the samples from all centres were assayed at the same time.

SHBG concentrations were measured as described by Bergink *et al.*[6]. HDL fractions were prepared using the phosphotungstate/magnesium chloride sedimentation method of Burnstein *et al.*[7]. Total cholesterol and triglycerides were determined using the Boehringer test method.

The measured values of all laboratory parameters were replaced by their logarithms to obtain normally distributed data, and were subjected to an analysis of co-variance using baseline measurements as co-variates, employing Winer's repeated measures design[8]. Owing to this choice of design, only those patients for whom complete data were available at every time point could be included in the analysis.

RESULTS

208 women treated with Marvelon completed 931 cycles within the trial period. The age structure is shown in Table 1. Nearly 50% of

Table 1 Age distribution

Age (years)	Number (%)
<20	101 (48.6)
20–24	46 (22.1)
25–29	34 (16.3)
30–34	19 (9.1)
35–39	8 (3.8)
>39	0 (0.0)

the patients were less than 20 years old, a high proportion of whom were new pill users.

Contraceptive efficacy appeared to be good. There was only one pregnancy, despite a high incidence (8.3% of all cycles) of forgotten tablets. This pregnancy started in cycle 3 – the patient did not admit to any forgotten tablets but reported suffering mid-cycle diarrhoea and vomiting for several days whilst on holiday abroad.

Table 2 Incidence of withdrawal bleeding on Marvelon

Cycle	No. of women completing cycle	Women experiencing withdrawal bleeding (%)
3	145	91.2
6	117	97.5

Incidences of withdrawal and unscheduled bleeding are shown in Figure 1 and Table 2. In the majority of patients the amount of

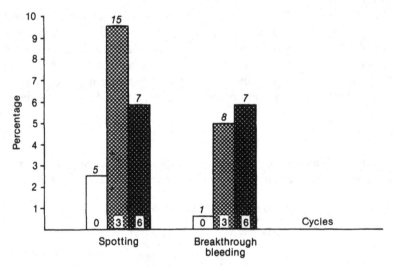

Figure 1 Incidence of unscheduled bleeding on Marvelon

withdrawal bleeding was the same or less than before treatment and the duration in days was also generally reduced. By cycle 6, 95% of withdrawal bleeds were starting between days 23 and 26.

40% of the unscheduled bleeding reported was experienced during the last 5 days of tablet taking. Only four patients found their

60

irregular bleeding sufficiently inconvenient to discontinue Marvelon treatment, and two of these dropped out during the first cycle. In more than 17% of all cycles in which unscheduled bleeding occurred, the patient reported forgetting between one and five tablets. However, during 60% of cycles in which one or two tablets were omitted, no unscheduled spotting or bleeding was reported.

No serious side-effects occurred. Various minor complaints were reported, both before and during treatment. The incidence of pre-treatment complaints together with those newly emergent complaints

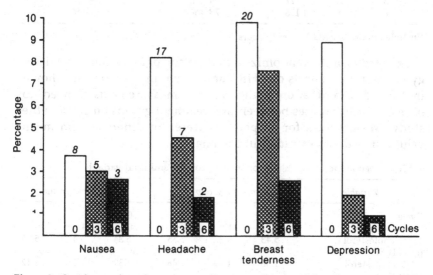

Figure 2 Incidence of newly emergent minor complaints on Marvelon

not recorded before treatment is shown in Figure 2. Fifteen patients withdrew from the trial as a result of side-effects, half of these during the first cycle. The only other complaint of interest was change in libido – a small number of women (< 5%) reporting either an increase or a decrease.

Table 3 Changes in blood pressure during Marvelon treatment

Cycle		Average deviation from pre-treatment cycle values (mm Hg)	
	No. of women	Systolic	Diastolic
3	127	−3.0	−1.2
6	118	−4.0	−1.9

Blood pressure and body weight changes are shown in Tables 3 and 4. Although the data is limited, effects on blood pressure were apparently minimal. A small weight increase is evident, but half of the trial patients were less than 20 years old and therefore still have growth potential.

Table 4 Changes in body weight during Marvelon treatment

Cycle	No. of women	No change, No. (%)	Average change from pre-treatment cycle (kg)
3	127	99 (78)	+0.5*
6	118	78 (66.1)	+0.8*

*Includes patients aged under 20 years.

The results of the randomized comparison of Marvelon and Microgynon and their effects on SHBG and serum lipoproteins are shown in Table 5. Examination of the baseline measurements showed no observable differences between the treatment groups on entry to the study. Mean values for all patients were not different from mean values of patients included in the analysis.

Table 5 Geometric mean values for serum proteins and lipid variables

Variable	Marvelon group			Microgynon group		
Cycle	0	3	6	0	3	6
No. of women	40	34	27	30	24	20
Total cholesterol ($mmol\,l^{-1}$)	5.43	6.27	5.55	5.34	5.47	5.03
HDL cholesterol ($mmol\,l^{-1}$)	1.38	1.63	1.46	1.39	1.33	1.12
Triglycerides ($mmol\,l^{-1}$)	0.73	1.02	1.08	0.80	0.80	0.80
SHBG ($nmol\,l^{-1}$)	69	187	184	63	71	64

HDL = High-density lipoprotein; SHBG = Serum hormone binding globulin.

There was no difference between treatments on effect on total cholesterol – both groups experienced a transient rise which had returned to pre-treatment values by 6 months. However, there were significant differences in HDL cholesterol values ($p \leqslant 0.0001$) between treatment groups. In the Marvelon-treated group the changes paralleled those seen in total cholesterol, with a transient rise at 3 months. In the Microgynon-treated group there was no change at 3 months but HDL-cholesterol levels had fallen considerably by 6 months.

Triglyceride levels were higher ($p \leqslant 0.005$) in the Marvelon treatment group.

SHBG levels were significantly increased ($p \leqslant 0.0001$) in the Marvelon-treated group as compared with the Microgynon group.

The effect of smoking was examined in relation to each parameter, but no significant differences between smokers and non-smokers could be found.

DISCUSSION

Extensive trials in Europe with the combination of 150 μg desogestrel and 30 μg ethinyloestradiol have yielded a Pearl Index for tablet failure of 0.0 and for patient failure[2] of 0.1. It was therefore unexpected to find a pregnancy in a small trial, although this patient's prolonged diarrhoea and vomiting may have resulted in malabsorption of the hormones.

The incidence of unscheduled bleeding during oral contraceptive use is known to decrease considerably during the first six cycles. By following up the patients for only six cycles it must be realized that a higher level of bleeding disturbances will be seen and should not therefore be compared with results of longer trials expressed as a percentage of total cycles. However, spotting and breakthrough bleeding were more common in this trial than in larger trials with Marvelon[2] where less than 5% spotting and 4.3% breakthrough bleeding were reported at six cycles. The data of this study were compatible with similar studies in Scandinavia[9,10].

The irregular bleeding reported in this trial was often during the last few days of pill taking and was closely related to a high incidence of forgotten pills. Despite this, it was encouraging to notice that on more than half the occasions when a patient forgot one or two tablets in a cycle there was no spotting or breakthrough bleeding.

Marvelon appeared to be well tolerated with respect to the common pill-induced side-effects and only a small proportion of patients discontinued the trial for reasons related to the treatment.

It is well known that a multiplicity of factors affect serum proteins and lipid levels[11]. Most studies have therefore been performed on volunteers, but this trial was conducted on routine clinic patients. Every reasonable effort was made to control for time of cycle and smoking habits were recorded. Allocation to treatment was according to a random list and assays were performed 'blind' in one laboratory.

Considerable interest has been generated in recent years as to the possibility of finding an oral contraceptive that might confer beneficial long-term effects by elevating HDL-cholesterol fractions[12]. Oestrogens are known to cause elevation of HDL-cholesterol values whilst progestogens commonly oppose this effect. In this trial a transient rise in HDL-cholesterol level was reported similar to that found in Scandinavian trials[3,4], compared with a fall in the Microgynon-treated group. The clinical relevance of these changes in the long term must remain unclear until epidemiological studies have been undertaken.

It has been suggested that an oral contraceptive that raised SHBG would confer advantages to women who suffer androgen-related side-effects such as hirsutism and acne[13]. This trial confirmed that Marvelon increases SHBG significantly, compared both with pre-treatment levels and Microgynon treatment. Although specific trials in acne and hirsutism would be desirable, it may well be that Marvelon would be a reasonable alternative to a levonorgestrel-containing pill in susceptible patients.

CONCLUSION

Preliminary experience of 12 British family planning clinics confirmed the choice of Marvelon as a useful new combined pill with minimal side-effects and potentially beneficial metabolic effects.

Acknowledgements

The author thanks his medical, nursing and administrative colleagues, without whom the study would not have been feasible; Dr W. Bergink for laboratory estimations; and Ir. J. Voerman and Mr D. Nelson for statistical analysis. The study was supported by Organon Laboratories Ltd.

References

1. Bergink, E. W., Hamburger, A. D., De Jager, E. and van der Vies, J. (1981). Binding of a contraceptive progestogen Org 2969 and its metabolites to receptor proteins and human sex hormone binding globulin. *J. Steroid Biochem.*, **14**, 175
2. Weijers, M. J. (1982). Clinical trial of an oral contraceptive containing 150 μg desogestrel and 30 μg ethinyloestradiol. *Clin. Ther.*, **4**, 359
3. Samsioe, G. (1982). Comparative effects of the oral contraceptive combinations

0.0150 mg desogestrel + 0.030 mg ethinyloestradiol and 0.150 mg levonorgestrel + 0.030 mg ethinyloestradiol on lipid and lipoprotein metabolism in healthy female volunteers. *Contraception*, **25**, 487

4. Bergink, E. W., Borglin, N. E., Klottrup, P. and Liukko, P. (1982). Effects of desogestrel and levonorgestrel in low-dose oestrogen oral contraceptives on serum lipoproteins. *Contraception*, **25**, 477

5. Gordon, T., Castelli, W. P. and Njortland, M. (1977). HDL as a protective factor against CHD – The Framingham study. *Am. J. Med.*, **62**, 707

6. Bergink, E. W., Holma, P. and Pyorala, T. (1981). Effects of oral contraceptive combinations containing levonorgestrel or desogestrel on serum proteins and androgen binding. *Scand. J. Clin. Lab. Invest.*, **41**, 663

7. Burstein, M., Scholnik, H. R. and Morfin, R. (1978). Rapid method for the isolation of lipoproteins from human serum by precipitation with polyanions. *J. Lipid. Res.*, **11**, 583

8. Winer, B. J. (1971). *Statistical Principles in Experimental Design*. (New York: McGraw Hill)

9. Borglin, N. E., Christensen, O. J. E., Culberg, G. *et al.* (1982). Scandinavian trial of an oral contraceptive containing 0.150 mg desogestrel and 0.03 mg ethinyloestradiol. *Acta Obstet. Gynecol. Scand. Suppl.*, **111**, 39

10. Culberg, G., Samsioe, G., Andersen, R. F., *et al.* (1982). Two oral contraceptives, efficacy, serum proteins and lipid metabolism. *Contraception*, **26**, 229

11. Bradley, D. D., Wingerd, J., Petitti, D. B., *et al.* (1978). Serum high density lipoproteins cholesterol in women using oral contraceptives, estrogens and progestins. *N. Engl. J. Med.*, **299**, 17

12. Kay, C. R. (1980). The happiness pill? *J. R. Coll. Gen. Pract.*, **30**, 8

13. el Makzangy, M. N., Wynn, V. and Lawrence, D. M. (1979). Sex hormone binding globulin capacity as an index of oestrogenicity or androgenicity in women on oral contraceptive steroids. *Clin. Endocrinol.*, **10**, 39

Index